The Keto Diet Weight Loss Book

Delicious and Easy-Going Recipes for Family
and Friends incl. KD-Planner to Lose Weight

Kate A. Taylor

ISBN-9798749783568

TABLE OF CONTENTS

Dinner

Snacks & Desserts

INTRODUCTION

WHAT IS THE KETOGENIC DIET?

A ketogenic diet consists of eating foods higher in fats and lower in carbohydrates than a typical diet. The diet also includes moderate protein consumption and is similar to other low-carb diets, such as the Atkins diet. A keto diet is especially useful for losing excess body fat, reducing hunger, and improving type 2 diabetes or metabolic syndrome. This book will help you learn how to get started with a ketogenic diet and includes over 50 recipes of all your favourite keto-friendly meals. As a bonus, a simple 14-day keto diet plan is included to help you achieve weight loss.

Ketogenic diets were originally developed to treat epilepsy in children whose seizures were treatment-resistant. It is understood that the brain needs energy from glucose to create a seizure. By following a ketogenic diet, the body is tricked into a state of fasting or starvation. In this state, the body uses fat instead of carbohydrates to create energy. When you feed the body more fats than carbohydrates, the liver creates ketones which the brain uses for energy instead of glucose from carbohydrates. There has been research that suggests a ketogenic diet reduces the frequency in seizures in some cases of childhood epilepsy.

From the success of the ketogenic diet for epilepsy, the diet has been popularised by mainstream media and followed by thousands for weight loss, diabetes, and to manage several other conditions explored in the following sections.

Glossary

Glucose - A type of sugar our bodies convert to energy

Carbohydrates - Complex sugars or starches

Ketosis - The process in which our body burns fats instead of glucose from carbohydrates to produce energy.

Ketones - The molecules created when our livers break down fat stores instead of carbohydrates to produce energy, during ketosis.

BENEFITS OF THE KETOGENIC DIET

Ketosis is normal evolutionary response humans have relied upon to survive periods of famine. Lab-carb diets work by stimulating this process which is why the ketogenic diet is so effective for weight loss and controlling blood sugar. Not only does the ketogenic diet work to help you shed pounds but also to keep the weight off in the long term. However, the long term success depends on how well you switch and stick to healthy and balanced dietary habits.

On a ketogenic diet, your entire body switches its fuel supply to run mostly on fat. When insulin levels drop very low, fat burning can increase dramatically. It becomes easier to access your fat stores to burn them off. This is great if you're trying to lose weight, but there are other benefits to following a ketogenic diet. You will feel less hunger and more energised. No more crashing after a sugar rush which often occurs when eating high-carb meals. Instead, you stay alert and focused for longer. A ketogenic diet also helps you to maintain a state of ketosis enabling you to enjoy the benefits of fasting - including weight loss - without having to fast long term.

Benefits of A Ketogenic Diet
- Reduces appetite.
- Easy weight loss.
- Less hunger pangs.
- Fat loss.
- Lowers blood fats.
- Increases good cholesterol.
- Improves bad cholesterol levels.
- Reduces blood sugar and insulin levels.
- Lowers blood pressure.
- Reduces risk of obesity.
- Reduces epileptic seizures.

WHO CAN FOLLOW THE KETOGENIC DIET?

You may be wondering if the ketogenic diet is safe as it contradicts common nutritional advice to follow a healthy, balanced diet which includes fats, carbohydrates and protein. To follow the keto diet you will have to replace foods rich loaded with carbohydrates with foods rich in fat and protein. If you plan to continue the diet for an extended period of time there are few things you should be aware of to ensure you continue to do what is right for your body.

The ketogenic diet could cause complications for anyone with blood sugar management issues. If you are diabetic, particularly with type 1 diabetes, or have a kidney disease you should consult your GP before making any changes to your diet. Those taking medication for high blood pressure and are pregnant or breastfeeding should also consult their healthcare provider before starting a keto diet.

An increased intake of high fat foods will likely increase your saturated fat intake. The UK National Health Service's (NHS) recommended daily fat intake is 30g for men, 20g for women, and children should have much less fat in their diet.

If you are considering switching your child to a ketogenic diet, please consult your paediatrician. They can ensure the diet is carefully balanced specifically for your child and can recommend the vitamins and other supplements necessary for their growing bodies.

Whilst you are following a ketogenic diet, your body is in a state of ketosis which is associated with some temporary symptoms that typically occur due to dehydration. These may include dry mouth, bad breath, headache, fatigue and nausea. Be sure to drink plenty of water and consider adapting your workout regime.

As the ketogenic diet restricts your intake of carbohydrates, a lower intake of dietary may have a negative impact on gut health. To ensure you maintain a healthy presence of gut-friendly bacteria, make sure you consume plenty of gut friendly foods like leafy greens, fermented vegetables and certain fats containing fatty acids like butter to support your gut.

HOW TO FOLLOW A KETOGENIC DIET

Foods that are generally allowed in a ketogenic diet include high-fat meats, fish, oils, nuts, high-fat dairy such as cheese, and low-carb vegetables such as leafy greens. Reducing carb levels can easily be achieved by cutting out bread, pasta, rice and other baked goods. However, to achieve a low level of carbs also means avoiding legumes, root vegetables, most fruits and starchy vegetables, such as potatoes.

Keto For Weight Loss

The Ketogenic diet is one of the most effective ways to lose weight quickly. Activating the process of ketosis is a natural way to lose weight and maintain a healthy body weight. Following a diet will not only improve your eating habits, but will also help you to better track the nutritional content of your meals. These skills along with routine physical activity will help to fast track your weight loss.

When following a ketogenic diet, focus on exercises that target fat cells. For example, practice cardiovascular exercises on a daily basis or workout at an intensity you are unable to keep a conversation going for at least 30 minutes, 5 days a week. Regular exercise whilst dieting will boost your metabolism and stimulate the leptin hormone that regulates your appetite. Also include weight resistance exercises to your workout regime. Lifting weights helps to burn off fat cells whilst maintaining muscle tone and strength.

Successfully losing weight whilst on a ketogenic diet requires a dedicated effort to make long-lasting changes to your lifestyle. If you are not losing as much weight as you hoped, look out for these common mistakes:

Excess calories - The most common mistake made when starting a ketogenic diet is eating too much. Counting calories whilst on a ketogenic diet is not necessary but general weight loss efforts require you to burn more calories than you consume. If you instead consume more calories than you burn the excess calories will be stored as body fat which works against your weight loss efforts.

Not enough calories - Whilst the most effective way to lose weight is to create a calorie deficit, if you do not consume enough calories by under-eating your metabolism will slow down and prevent you from losing weight. If the body is not supplied with enough calories, it begins to burn calories as slowly as possible to save energy. Too few calories can also lead to other health issues, such as anemia, hair loss, loss of menstrual periods, irregular heart beats, and mental health issues.

Impatience - To make any long-lasting changes to your lifestyle takes time. It also takes time for the body to switch from converting glucose from carbohydrates to burning fat for energy. At the start of a ketogenic diet, your body must first burn excess glucose before entering a state of ketosis and begin burning fat for fuel. Be patient with yourself and your body. Typically, it takes 2-6 days to enter a state of ketosis but this is dependent on many different factors and will differ from person to person. For people who usually eat a high-carb diet it can take them a week or longer for their bodies to reach a state of ketosis.

Food allergies - Even if you are allergic or intolerant to nuts, milk, eggs, fish, seafood or shellfish, you may gain weight whilst on a ketogenic diet. Food allergies and sensitivities can cause digestive problems and inflammation which can lead to an increase in body weight due to fat deposits, excess water and other issues. Also, if you are leptin resistant, you may find it difficult to lose weight whilst following a ketogenic diet. Stress, overeating and calorie restrictions can trigger a leptin response.

Constant dehydration - Most people are completely unaware that they are not drinking enough and are dehydrated. Ensuring you are adequately hydrated is important as it ensures many important bodily processes, such as digestion, mood, and nutrient absorption, are functioning optimally. Drinking enough water is vital to your overall health.

In this book, we have included a bonus ketogenic diet weight loss meal planner. It gives you 14 days worth or suggested meals for breakfast, lunch, and dinner. Taking out the guesswork of what to eat every day will save you time with food preparation and you will be more likely to stick with the diet.

Overview Of The Ketogenic Diet

70-75% fats

20% protein

5-10% carbs

Once you have achieved your healthy, ideal weight, you can slightly increase the amount of carbohydrates you consume. Be sure to continue to track your calorie intake and follow the ketogenic diet regularly. You can try rotating low-carb days with moderate-carb and high-carb days.

If you are interested in following a ketogenic diet you should consult your GP. Before getting started with the diet, eat liver-supportive foods like garlic and onions and avoid sugar, caffeine and alcohol.

The key to success on a ketogenic diet is consuming good fats. The ketogenic diet promotes monounsaturated and polyunsaturated fats that can lower your risk for heart disease, and reduce triglyceride levels. Fatty fish such as salmon, mackerel, and sardines are great sources of omega-3 fatty acids. Choose coconut oil, olive oil, nuts, seeds, and avocado that increase good HDL (High-density lipoprotein). Below is a handy list of foods you are encouraged to eat and which foods to avoid whilst on a ketogenic diet.

What To Eat And Avoid Whilst On The Ketogenic Diet

Allowed
- Meat: Beef, lamb, chicken, pork, chicken, turkey, etc. Grass-fed is best.
- Fish: Salmon, sardines, cod, trout, haddock, etc. Wild-caught fish is best.
- Eggs: Omega-3-enriched or pastured eggs are best.
- Vegetables: Spinach, kale, cauliflower, broccoli, carrots, etc.

- Fruits: Apples, blueberries, strawberries, raspberries, oranges, pears.
- Nuts and seeds: Almonds, walnuts, hemp seeds, sunflower seeds, etc.
- High-fat dairy: Cheese, butter, yogurt, heavy cream.
- Tubers: Potatoes and sweet potatoes.
- Unrefined grains: Brown rice, quinoa, oats, etc.
- Legumes: Lentils, pinto beans, chickpeas, black beans, etc.
- Fats and oils: Butter, coconut oil, lard, ghee, olive oil and fish oils.
- Drinks: Water, tea, coffee, red wine.

Avoid
- Sugar: Soft drinks, fruit juices, sweets, agave, ice cream and other products containing added sugar.
- Refined grains: Wheat, rice, bread, cereal and pasta, barley and rye.
- Trans fats: Hydrogenated or partially hydrogenated oils.
- Diet and low-fat products: Most fat-reduced dairy products, cereals or crackers contain added sugar.
- Highly processed foods
- Starchy vegetables

EASY KETO SUBSTITUTES

Following a diet should be easy enough to follow and filled with delicious meals your friends and family will enjoy. Advancements in food technology and food science have brought keto-friendly versions of almost every common product. Converting a recipe to a keto meal may be as simple as finding a keto-friendly substitute for certain ingredients. Even restaurants and ready-meals are offering keto options. However, these product substitutions can be expensive and can be easily made at home.

Here are some handy keto substitutes to try when recreating your favourite meals:

Pasta – You can spiralize zucchini, cucumber or pumpkin and eat them with

your favorite keto sauce, melted cheese or fried eggs. Otherwise, you can

purchase keto pasta such as kelp noodles and shirataki noodles.

Baked goods, pizza, and bread – Low-carb cheese rolls, roasted eggplant rounds or grilled

portobello mushrooms are great alternatives to burger buns and bread. You can easily warm them and fill them with your favorite fillings. For pizza and flatbread, you can use cauliflower, almond meal, coconut flour, or ground nuts. Refined bread is low in micronutrients, high in carbs, and generally bad for your health. Some good alternatives include nori sheets and cloud bread. You will find great keto desserts to replace your usual baked goods. For pancakes, tortillas, and wraps, simply mix almond flour with milk, eggs, chia seeds, or flax meal. Other ideas include kale, cabbage leaves, lettuce leaves, zucchini to hold fillings.

Snacks – You will find so many snack recipes in this book and there are plenty more to enjoy whilst on the ketogenic diet. You can make veggie crisps using zucchini, Brussels sprouts, or kale. You can use pork rinds and cheese to make breadsticks.

Fried foods – As an alternative to breadcrumbs you can use pork rinds, psyllium husk, and grated parmesan to make a good coating for fish, chicken tenders and fritters.

Other keto substitutes – Cauliflower rice is a popular side dish on the ketogenic diet but you can also make casseroles, salads, curries, and stews. As for keto sushi, wrap sashimi and cauliflower rice in nori sheets. Oatmeal and granola are great for porridge or cereal, you can make them with nuts, seeds, milk, and butter.

Tips For Switching To A Ketogenic Diet
- Reduce carbs.
- Get plenty of protein.
- Add fat for flavour and to support your gut.
- Track your fat intake using a keto diet tracker or app.
- Eat one piece of fruit per day.
- Avoid overeating cheese and nuts.
- Eat plenty of leafy greens.
- Read the ingredients lists.
- Eat dark chocolate in moderation.
- Drink alcohol in moderation.
- Avoid caffeine.

RECIPES

BREAKFAST

HARD-BOILED EGGS WITH AVOCADO

Time: 10 mins | Serves 4

Net carbs: 5.7g | Fat: 17.6g

Protein: 12.2g | Kcal: 222

INGREDIENTS

- 8 eggs
- 2 avocados, pitted and sliced
- 1/2 teaspoon dried dill weed
- 1 tablespoon lemon juice
- 1/2 teaspoon kosher salt

INSTRUCTIONS

1   Add the eggs and water (2.5cm above the eggs) to a saucepan and bring to a boil.
2   Remove from heat and let it sit for 15 minutes.
3   Peel the eggs and slice them into halves.
4   Sprinkle the eggs with salt and dill.
5   Serve topped with avocado slices and fresh lemon juice.

BREAKFAST EGG SALAD

Time: 15 mins | Serves 4
Net carbs: 6.8g | Fat: 37.1g
Protein: 28g | Kcal: 474

INGREDIENTS

- 4 eggs
- 1 cucumber, sliced
- 4 cups lettuce, broken into pieces
- 1 avocado, pitted, peeled and sliced
- 240g goat cheese, crumbled

INSTRUCTIONS

1. Heat 2 tablespoons of canola oil in a frying pan over the highest heat.

2. Crack the eggs into the oil and fry them for 1 to 2 minutes or until the yolks are set, then set aside.

3. Mix the cucumber and lettuce in a serving bowl.

4. Place fried eggs and avocado on top.

5. Garnish with crumbled cheese and serve.

SKINNY EGGS WITH SPINACH

Time: 10 mins | Serves 4

Net carbs: 3.3g | Fat: 13.1g

Protein: 12.9g | Kcal: 183

INGREDIENTS

- 8 eggs, well whisked
- 2 teaspoons olive oil
- 1/2 teaspoon garlic powder
- Sea salt and cayenne pepper, to taste
- 150g baby spinach

INSTRUCTIONS

1 Heat the olive oil in a cast-iron skillet over medium-high heat.
2 Add in the baby spinach and garlic powder; season with salt and cayenne pepper and cook for 1 to 2 minutes or until wilted.
3 Fold in the eggs, and continue to cook, stirring continuously with a spatula.
4 Serve while hot.

FRITTATA WITH MEDITERRANEAN HERBS

Time: 30 mins | Serves 4

Net carbs: 6.1g | Fat: 30.5g

Protein: 23.1g | Kcal: 394

INGREDIENTS

- 6 eggs
- 60g bacon, chopped
- 1 teaspoon Mediterranean herbs
- 25g red onion, peeled and sliced
- 240g Feta cheese, crumbled

INSTRUCTIONS

1 Preheat the oven to 180 degrees Celsius.
2 Brush a baking pan with a nonstick spray.
3 Mix the eggs, bacon, herbs and onion until well combined.
4 Season with salt and black pepper.
5 Pour the mixture into the prepared baking dish.
6 Bake for 15 minutes until the eggs are set.
7 Crumble feta cheese over the top and continue to bake for 5 minutes more.
8 Serve while hot.

BREAKFAST SAUSAGE AND CHEESE BITES

Time: 20 mins | Serves 4

Net carbs: 4.7g | Fat: 34.6g

Protein: 19.6g | Kcal: 412

INGREDIENTS

- 150g breakfast sausage
- 65g almond flour
- 115g cheddar cheese, shredded
- 4 tablespoons mozzarella cheese, freshly grated
- 2 eggs

INSTRUCTIONS

1. Preheat your oven to 180 degrees Celsius.
2. Thoroughly combine all ingredients until everything is well mixed.
3. Roll the mixture into balls.
4. Place the balls on a parchment-lined baking pan sheet.
5. Bake in the preheated oven for about 15 to 17 minutes.
6. Serve while hot.

SOUFFLÉ WITH SAUSAGE AND CHEESE

Time: 55 mins | Serves 8
Net carbs: 4.5g | Fat: 28.7g
Protein: 17.6g | Kcal: 348

INGREDIENTS

- 240g Chorizo sausage, sliced
- 4 scallions, chopped
- 240g cream cheese
- 10 eggs
- 1 cup Swiss cheese, grated

INSTRUCTIONS

1. Preheat an oven-proof skillet over a moderate flame.
2. Brown the sausage for 5 minutes, breaking apart it with a wide spatula.
3. Stir in the scallions and continue to sauté for a further 3 minutes.
4. Season with salt and black pepper.
5. In a mixing dish, combine the cream cheese and eggs.
6. Pour the egg mixture into the oven-proof skillet.
7. Transfer the skillet to the preheated oven.
8. Bake at 180 degrees Celsius for about 30 minutes.
9. Top with Swiss cheese and continue to bake for 7 minutes more or until the cheese is hot and bubbly.
10. Serve while hot.

CLASSIC KETO MUFFINS

Time: 20 mins | Serves 4

Net carbs: 5.4g | Fat: 23.1g

Protein: 16.4g | Kcal: 292

INGREDIENTS

- 120g cheddar cheese, shredded
- 6 tablespoons almond flour
- 2 tablespoons flaxseed meal
- 4 eggs
- 1/4 teaspoon baking soda

INSTRUCTIONS

1 Preheat the oven to 180 degrees Celsius.
2 Thoroughly combine all of the above ingredients until well mixed.
3 Coat a muffin pan with cupcake liners.
4 Spoon the batter into the muffin pan.
5 Bake in the preheated oven for 16 minutes.
6 Place on a wire rack for 10 minutes before unmolding and serving.
7 Serve with eggs.

BREAKFAST BACON AND KALE MUFFINS

Time: 25 mins | Serves 4
Net carbs: 5.1g | Fat: 29.8g
Protein: 24g | Kcal: 384

INGREDIENTS

- 230g bacon
- 20g kale
- 8g tomato paste with garlic and onion
- 6 eggs
- 85g Grana Padano cheese, shredded

INSTRUCTIONS

1. Preheat your oven to 190 degrees Celsius.
2. Cook the bacon for 3 to 4 minutes over the highest setting, then set aside.
3. Add in the kale, tomato paste, eggs and Grana Padano cheese.
4. Add in the bacon.
5. Spoon the batter into lightly greased muffin cups; then, bake for 15 minutes or until the edges are golden brown.
6. Serve while hot.

CHEESY MINI FRITTATAS WITH SAUSAGE

Time: 35 mins | Serves 6
Net carbs: 1.9g | Fat: 23.7g
Protein: 16.1g | Kcal: 287

INGREDIENTS

- 5 eggs
- 80g double cream
- 200g pork sausage, sliced
- 1 bell pepper, chopped
- 100g goat cheese, crumbled

INSTRUCTIONS

1 Start by preheating your oven to 180 degrees Celsius.
2 Cook the sausage and bell pepper in a preheated nonstick pan over a moderate heat.
3 In a mixing bowl, combine the eggs and double cream; stir in the pepper/sausage mixture. Season with salt and black pepper.
4 Spoon the mixture into foil-lined muffin cups and bake for approximately 20 minutes.
5 Top with goat cheese and bake for about 6 minutes or until slightly browned around the edges. Serve while hot.

BROCCOLI CHEESE PIE

Time: 30 mins | Serves 4

Net carbs: 5.3g | Fat: 23.2g

Protein: 19.2g | Kcal: 308

INGREDIENTS

- ◆ 2 teaspoons olive oil
- ◆ 6 eggs
- ◆ 1 red onion, sliced
- ◆ 6 tablespoons Greek yoghurt
- ◆ 140g broccoli florets
- ◆ 115g cheddar cheese, shredded

INSTRUCTIONS

1. Heat 2 teaspoons of olive oil in an oven-safe skillet over medium-high heat.
2. Sweat red onion and broccoli until they have softened or about 4 minutes.
3. Season with salt and black pepper.
4. In a mixing bowl, whisk Greek yoghurt and eggs until well mixed.
5. Scrape the mixture into the pan.
6. Bake at 180 degrees Celsius for 15 to 20 minutes or until a toothpick inserted into a muffin comes out dry and clean.
7. Top with cheddar cheese and bake for 5 to 6 minutes more.
8. Serve while hot.

DEVILED EGGS WITH TUNA

Time: 15 mins | Serves 4

Net carbs: 2.3g | Fat: 4.7g

Protein: 14.5g | Kcal: 112

INGREDIENTS

- 4 eggs
- 1 can tuna, drained
- 1/2 red onions, chopped
- 4 teaspoons cottage cheese, room temperature
- 1 tablespoon Dijon mustard

INSTRUCTIONS

1. In a saucepan, bring the eggs and water to a boil.
2. Switch the heat off and let cool for about 10 minutes.
3. Peel away the shells and separate the egg whites and yolks.
4. Mash the yolks with tuna, onions, cheese, and mustard.
5. Sprinkle with the salt and black pepper, if desired.
6. Divide the mixture among egg whites and serve well chilled.

SWISS CHEESE AND ONION SOUP

Time: 15 mins | Serves 2

Net carbs: 6.6g | Fat: 27.2g

Protein: 21g | Kcal: 365

INGREDIENTS

- 2 tablespoons ghee, at room temperature
- 80g shallots, chopped
- 125ml cream of onion soup
- 250g yogurt
- 120g Swiss cheese, shredded

INSTRUCTIONS

1. Melt the ghee in a heavy-bottomed pot over medium-high flame.
2. Sauté the shallots for about 4 minutes or until tender.
3. Pour in the cream of onion soup along with 125 ml of water.
4. Reduce the heat to simmer.
5. Cook for 10 to 12 minutes or until heated through.
6. Remove from heat and stir in the yogurt and Swiss cheese.
7. Mix until everything is thoroughly combined.
8. Serve while hot.

MEDITERRANEAN TOMATO FRITTATA

Time: 25 mins | Serves 4

Net carbs: 3.4g | Fat: 22.4g

Protein: 19.6g | Kcal: 299

INGREDIENTS

- 6 eggs
- 80g Greek-style yoghurt
- 2 scallions, chopped
- 1 tomato, sliced
- 160g cheddar cheese, shredded

INSTRUCTIONS

1 Preheat your oven to 180 degrees Celsius.
2 Butter a pie pan and set it aside.
3 Thoroughly combine the Greek-style yoghurt and scallions.
4 Spoon the mixture into the prepared pan.
5 Top with the tomato slices.
6 Scatter the cheese over the top.
7 Bake for about 30 minutes or until the edges appear cooked.
8 Slice into four wedges and serve.

CHEESY SPANISH TORTILLA

Time: 30 mins | Serves 4

Net carbs: 5.2g | Fat: 24.2g

Protein: 20.2g | Kcal: 324

INGREDIENTS

- 125g leeks, chopped
- 1 Spanish pepper, chopped
- 60ml milk
- 5 eggs, beaten
- 225g Mozzarella cheese, shredded

INSTRUCTIONS

1 Melt 1 tablespoon of butter in a saucepan over medium-high flame.
2 Cook the leeks and Spanish pepper until they have softened.
3 Season with salt and freshly ground black pepper.
4 Spoon the sautéed mixture into a buttered baking pan.
5 In a bowl, whisk the milk and eggs until pale and frothy.
6 Pour the mixture into the prepared baking pan.
7 Top with Mozzarella cheese and bake in the preheated oven at 180 degrees Celsius for 23 to 25 minutes.
8 Let it cool on a wire rack for about 10 minutes before cutting and serving.

HERBED CHEESE BALL

Time: 10 mins | Serves 10

Net carbs: 2g | Fat: 15.7g

Protein: 7.2g | Kcal: 176

INGREDIENTS

- 125g sour cream
- 240g cheddar cheese, shredded
- 150g cream cheese, softened
- 2 tablespoons mayonnaise
- 1 tablespoon Moroccan herb mix

INSTRUCTIONS

1. Thoroughly combine the sour cream, cheddar cheese, cream cheese, and mayonnaise.
2. Cover the mixture with a plastic wrap and place in your refrigerator for about 3 hours.
3. Roll the mixture over Moroccan herb mix until well coated.
4. Serve with assorted keto veggies.

LUNCH

CLASSIC FAMILY CHEESEBURGERS

Time: 15 mins | Serves 4
Net carbs: 4.8g | Fat: 35.1g
Protein: 46g | Kcal: 533

INGREDIENTS

- 500g ground beef
- 3 slices cheddar cheese
- 1 tablespoon olive oil
- 1 white onion, sliced
- 1 teaspoon burger seasoning mix

INSTRUCTIONS

1. With oiled hands, mix the ground beef with the burger seasoning mix.
2. Season with salt and black pepper to taste.
3. Roll the mixture into 4 equal patties.
4. Heat the olive oil in a grill pan over medium-high heat.
5. Grill the burgers for 5 to 6 minutes, flipping them over with a wide spatula.
6. Top with cheese and cook for 5 minutes more or until cheese has melted.
7. Serve with onions.

CHICKEN THIGH SALAD

Time: 20 mins | Serves 2
Net carbs: 6.7g | Fat: 29g
Protein: 3.7g | Kcal: 456

INGREDIENTS

- 2 chicken thighs, skinless
- 1 tablespoon Dijon mustard
- 1 tablespoon red wine vinegar
- 60g mayonnaise
- 2 spring onion stalks, chopped
- ½ head Romaine lettuce, torn into pieces

INSTRUCTIONS

1 In a preheated skillet, cook the chicken thighs until crunchy on the outside.
2 Discard the bones and transfer the meat to a salad bowl.
3 Add Dijon mustard.
4 Stir in the other ingredients.
5 Serve chilled.

FAJITA WITH ZUCCHINI

Time: 20 mins | Serves 4

Net carbs: 5.6g | Fat: 9.2g

Protein: 26g | Kcal: 212

INGREDIENTS

- 2 tablespoons olive oil
- 1 red onion, sliced
- 1 teaspoon Fajita seasoning mix
- 500g turkey breasts
- 1 zucchini, spiralized
- 1 chilli pepper, chopped
- 8g salsa

INSTRUCTIONS

1 In a nonstick skillet, heat 1 tablespoon of olive oil over a medium-high flame.
2 Cook the turkey breasts for 6 to 7 minutes on each side.
3 Slice the meat into strips and set aside.
4 Heat another tablespoon of olive oil and sauté the onion and chilli pepper until they are just tender.
5 Sprinkle the Fajita seasoning mix.
6 Add in the zucchini and the turkey.
7 Cook for 4 minutes more or until everything is cooked through.
8 Serve with salsa.

SPICY PORK MEATBALLS

Time: 25 mins | Serves 4
Net carbs: 2.3g | Fat: 50.1g
Protein: 0.5g | Kcal: 557

INGREDIENTS

- 500g minced pork
- 5g scallions, chopped
- 100g bacon
- 1 garlic clove, minced
- 1 teaspoon taco seasoning blend

INSTRUCTIONS

1 Mix all ingredients until everything is well incorporated.
2 Shape the meat mixture into golf-ball-sized balls.
3 In a lightly greased nonstick skillet, sear the meatballs over medium-high heat until golden brown on all sides.
4 Serve while hot.

AUTUMN BUTTERNUT SQUASH STEW

Time: 35 mins | Serves 4
Net carbs: 6.8g | Fat: 11.5g
Protein: 2.5g | Kcal: 148

INGREDIENTS

- 2 tablespoons olive oil
- 1 Spanish onion, peeled and diced
- 250g butternut squash, diced
- 750ml water or vegetable broth
- 1 celery stalk, chopped
- 90g baby spinach
- 4 tablespoons sour cream

INSTRUCTIONS

1 Heat olive oil in a stock-pot over medium-high flame.
2 Sauté the Spanish onion until tender and fragrant.
3 Stir in the butternut squash and celery.
4 Pour in water or vegetable broth.
5 Reduce the temperature to medium-low and continue to cook for 25 to 30 minutes.
6 Fold in spinach, cover, and let it stand in the residual heat until the spinach leaves wilt.
7 Season with salt and black pepper to taste.
8 Serve with cold sour cream.

FRIED COD FILLETS

Time: 15 mins | Serves 4

Net carbs: 4.1g | Fat: 29.5g

Protein: 31.9g | Kcal: 406

INGREDIENTS

- 2 tablespoons butter
- 4 cod fillets
- 235g Parmesan cheese, preferably freshly grated
- 1 teaspoon dried rosemary, crushed
- 60g almond flour

INSTRUCTIONS

1 Place the fish, almond flour, salt, black pepper, and rosemary in a resealable bag.
2 Shake bag to coat well.
3 Press cod fillets into the grated Parmesan cheese.
4 Melt the butter in a nonstick skillet over medium-high heat.
5 Cook the fish until it is nearly opaque, about 5 minutes on each side.
6 Serve while hot.

EGGPLANT AND GOAT CHEESE BAKE

Time: 35 mins | Serves 4
Net carbs: 7.2g | Fat: 41.4g
Protein: 18.4g | Kcal: 477

INGREDIENTS

- 2 bell peppers, deveined and quartered
- 1 eggplant, cut into rounds
- 2 tablespoons olive oil
- 120g sour cream
- 360g goat cheese
- 2 vine-ripe tomatoes, sliced
- 1 teaspoon Asian spice mix

INSTRUCTIONS

1 Preheat your oven to 210 degrees Celsius.
2 Lightly oil a baking dish with a nonstick spray.
3 Place the peppers and eggplant into the baking dish.
4 Place the sliced tomatoes on top.
5 Drizzle 2 tablespoons of olive oil all over the vegetables.
6 Season with the Asian spice mix.
7 Bake in the preheated oven for 15 to 17 minutes.
8 Rotate the pan and continue to bake for a further 7 to 9 minutes.
9 Top with sour cream and cheese and serve.

ROASTED ASPARAGUS SALAD

Time: 20 mins | Serves 5
Net carbs: 7.7g | Fat: 11.5g
Protein: 3.5g | Kcal: 179

INGREDIENTS

- 2 tablespoons olive oil
- 750g asparagus spears, trimmed
- 150g cherry tomatoes, halved
- 3 tablespoons sour cream
- 5 tablespoons mayonnaise

INSTRUCTIONS

1. Toss the asparagus with olive oil and Italian seasoning mix.
2. Transfer to a roasting pan and roast at 210 degrees Celsius for about 15 minutes until crispy and lightly charred.
3. In a mixing dish, combine sour cream and mayonnaise.
4. Toss asparagus with this mixture and top with cherry tomatoes.
5. Serve.

ANCHOVIES WITH CAESAR DRESSING

Time: 15 mins | Serves 4
Net carbs: 1g | Fat: 34.4g
Protein: 32.6g | Kcal: 449

INGREDIENTS

- 6 anchovies, cleaned and deboned
- 2 egg yolks
- 1 teaspoon Dijon mustard
- 1 fresh garlic clove, peeled
- 80ml extra-virgin olive oil

INSTRUCTIONS

1. Rinse the anchovies and pat dry.
2. Grill the anchovies in a lightly greased grill pan just until golden.
3. Blend egg yolks, Dijon mustard, garlic, and extra-virgin olive oil until smooth and creamy.
4. Serve warm anchovies with the Caesar dressing and serve.

FISH AND EGG SALAD

Time: 20 mins | Serves 4
Net carbs: 3.5g | Fat: 19.3g
Protein: 26.5g | Kcal: 300

INGREDIENTS

- 500g red snapper fillets
- 5 eggs
- 140g lettuce salad
- 1 bell pepper, deseeded and sliced
- 1 tomato, sliced
- 4 tablespoons olive oil

INSTRUCTIONS

1 Steam the red snapper fillets for 8 to 10 minutes or until fork-tender.
2 Cut the fish into small strips.
3 Boil the eggs in a saucepan for about 9 minutes.
4 Peel the eggs and carefully slice them.
5 Place bell peppers, tomato, and lettuce leaves in a salad bowl.
6 Add in 4 tablespoons of olive oil and 4 tablespoons of apple cider vinegar. Toss to combine well.
7 Top with the reserved fish and eggs and salt to taste.
8 Serve well-chilled.

COD FISH SALAD

Time: 15 mins | Serves 5
Net carbs: 6.4g | Fat: 6.9g
Protein: 42.7g | Kcal: 276

INGREDIENTS

- 5 cod fillets
- 50g lettuce, cut into small pieces
- 60ml balsamic vinegar
- 1 red onion, sliced
- 75g green cabbage, shredded

INSTRUCTIONS

1 Heat 1 tablespoon of olive oil in a large saucepan over a moderate flame.
2 Once hot, cook the fish for about 10 minutes or until it is golden brown on
3 top.
4 Flake the fish, then set aside.
5 Whisk 3 tablespoons of olive oil and balsamic vinegar; season with salt and black pepper.
6 Combine the lettuce, green cabbage, and onion in a serving bowl.
7 Dress the salad and top with codfish, then serve.

SEA BASS IN DIJON SAUCE

Time: 20 mins | Serves 3

Net carbs: 1.4g | Fat: 23.2g

Protein: 24.2g | Kcal: 314

INGREDIENTS

- 3 sea bass fillets
- 2 tablespoons olive oil
- 3 tablespoons butter
- 2 cloves garlic, minced
- 1 tablespoon Dijon mustard

INSTRUCTIONS

1. Pat dry the sea bass fillets.
2. Heat olive oil in a frying pan over a medium-high flame.
3. Cook the fish fillets for 4 to 5 minutes on each side until they are opaque.
4. Season with red pepper and salt to taste.
5. In another saucepan, melt the butter over a low flame.
6. Sauté the garlic for 30 seconds.
7. Add in the mustard and continue to simmer for 2 to 3 minutes.
8. Serve warm fish fillets with Dijon sauce.

FISH CAKES WITH CLASSIC HORSERADISH SAUCE

Time: 20 mins | Serves 4
Net carbs: 1.9g | Fat: 8.3g
Protein: 27.3g | Kcal: 206

INGREDIENTS

- 500g cod fillets
- 8 tablespoons Ricotta cheese
- 4 tablespoons parmesan cheese, grated
- 1 teaspoon creamed horseradish
- 2 eggs, beaten

INSTRUCTIONS

1. Steam the cod fillets for about 10 minutes or until easily flaked with a fork.
2. Chop your fish and mix with eggs and parmesan cheese.
3. Form the mixture into 4 fish cakes. Heat 2 tablespoons of olive oil in a frying skillet.
4. Once hot, cook the fish cakes over medium-high heat for 3 to 4 minutes on each side.
5. Make the sauce by whisking Ricotta cheese and creamed horseradish.
6. Serve while hot.

SALMON LETTUCE TACOS

Time: 20 mins | Serves 5

Net carbs: 5.3g | Fat: 14.1g

Protein: 38.6g | Kcal: 304

INGREDIENTS

- 10 lettuce leaves
- 1kg salmon
- 1 tomato, halved
- 1 avocado, pitted and peeled
- 4 tablespoons green onions

INSTRUCTIONS

1. Toss the salmon with salt and black pepper to your liking.
2. Drizzle the salmon with 2 tablespoons of olive oil and grill over medium-high heat for about 15 minutes.
3. Flake the fish with two forks.
4. Divide the fish among the lettuce leaves.
5. Puree avocado, tomato, and green onions in your blender until your desired
6. consistency is reached.
7. Add 1 tablespoon of olive oil to your blender, if desired.
8. Top each taco with the avocado sauce, drizzle with fresh lemon juice and serve.

KETO MUSHROOM CHILLI

Time: 20 mins | Serves 3

Net carbs: 6g | Fat: 11.3g

Protein: 6.9g | Kcal: 159

INGREDIENTS

- 90g bacon, diced
- 375g brown mushrooms, sliced
- 2 cloves garlic, minced
- 1 brown onion, chopped
- 3 tablespoons dry red wine

INSTRUCTIONS

1   In a preheated soup pot, fry the bacon until crisp or about 4 minutes, then set aside.

2   In the pan drippings, sauté the brown mushrooms, garlic, and brown onion and until they have softened.

3   Pour in red wine and deglaze the pot with a wide spatula.

4   Add in 1 teaspoon of chilli powder.

5   Reduce the heat to simmer.

6   Stir in the remaining ingredients and continue cooking for 10 to 15 minutes or until the sauce has thickened.

7   Garnish with the reserved bacon and serve warm.

DINNER

SPAGHETTI BOLOGNESE

Time: 30 mins | Serves 4

Net carbs: 4g | Fat: 28.7g

Protein: 20.2g | Kcal: 357

INGREDIENTS

- 2 zucchinis, spiralised (zoodles)
- 2 medium-sized tomatoes, pureed
- 500g ground pork
- 3 teaspoons olive oil
- 2 cloves garlic, pressed

INSTRUCTIONS

1   In a frying pan, heat the oil over a moderate heat.
2   Cook minced pork for about 5 minutes or until browned.
3   Sauté the garlic for 30 seconds more.
4   Stir in the pureed tomatoes and bring to a boil.
5   Turn the heat to medium-low and let it simmer for a further 20 to 25 minutes.
6   Add in the zoodles and continue to simmer for 2 minutes more.
7   Serve while hot.

HEARTY BEEF AND VEGETABLE STEW

Time: 45 mins | Serves 4

Net carbs: 5.4g | Fat: 16.8g

Protein: 41g | Kcal: 372

INGREDIENTS

◆ 60g bacon, diced

◆ 60g herb pasta sauce, no sugar added

◆ 750g beef steak, boneless and cut into 1-1/2-inch pieces

◆ 1 parsnip, chopped

◆ 2 bell pepper, chopped

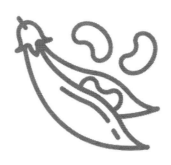

INSTRUCTIONS

1. In a Dutch oven, cook the bacon over medium-high heat, then set aside.
2. In the bacon grease, brown the beef pieces for about 4 minutes or until nicely browned, then set aside.
3. Sauté the parsnip and peppers for 4 minutes more until they have softened.
4. Season with salt and black pepper to taste.
5. Add in herb pasta sauce along with beef.
6. When the mixture reaches boiling, reduce the heat to simmer.
7. Simmer for about 30 minutes or until everything is thoroughly cooked.
8. Serve garnished with the bacon.

CLASSIC SUNDAY ROAST

Time: 55 mins | Serves 5

Net carbs: 0.7g | Fat: 20.6g

Protein: 51.1g | Kcal: 405

INGREDIENTS

- 1kg round rump beef
- 1 tablespoon pot roast seasoning mix
- 4 tablespoons olive oil
- 1 tablespoon prepared horseradish, strained
- 125ml beef stock

INSTRUCTIONS

1. Cut slits in the beef using a small knife.
2. In a mixing bowl, combine pot roast seasoning. olive oil, and horseradish.
3. Add the salt and black pepper to taste.
4. Let the roast sit in your refrigerator overnight.
5. Place the roast in a baking pan and pour in the beef stock.
6. Roast the beef in the preheated oven at 220 degrees Celsius for 30 minutes.
7. Lower the temperature to 170 degrees Celsius and roast for a further 11 to 16 minutes.
8. Serve while hot.

CHEESY ZUCCHINI LASAGNA

Time: 45 mins | Serves 7

Net carbs: 3.3g | Fat: 31.8g

Protein: 42g | Kcal: 467

INGREDIENTS

- ◆ 1 large-sized zucchini, sliced

- ◆ 1.5kg minced beef

- ◆ 7 eggs, whisked

- ◆ 1 shallot, chopped

- ◆ 1 tablespoon steak seasoning blend

- ◆ 120g Grana Padano cheese, shredded

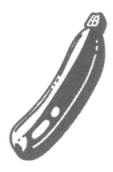

INSTRUCTIONS

1. Heat 2 tablespoons of olive oil in a saucepan over a medium-high flame.
2. Sear the minced beef for about 5 minutes.
3. Stir in the shallot and continue to cook for 3 to 4 minutes more or until it has softened.
4. Sprinkle with 1 tablespoon of the steak seasoning blend.
5. Spread 1/3 of the beef mixture on the bottom of a lightly greased baking dish.
6. Top with the layer of zucchini slices.
7. Repeat until you run out of the filling and zucchini.
8. Spoon the eggs over the top.
9. Top with the cheese and cover with a piece of foil.
10. Bake in the preheated oven at 190 degrees Celsius for 18 to 20 minutes.
11. Remove the aluminium foil and bake for a further 13 minutes until it is golden around the edges.
12. Serve while hot.

EASY CHICKEN CASSEROLE

Time: 30 mins | Serves 4

Net carbs: 6.2g | Fat: 1.5g

Protein: 50g | Kcal: 410

INGREDIENTS

- 2 ripe tomatoes, chopped
- 375g chicken breast fillets, chopped into bite-sized chunks
- 120g heavy whipping cream
- 2 garlic cloves, sliced
- 1/2 teaspoon Asian spice mix

INSTRUCTIONS

1. Preheat your oven to 190 degrees Celsius.
2. Spritz a casserole dish with nonstick spray.
3. Add the chicken, garlic, Asian spice mix to the casserole dish.
4. Top with tomatoes and heavy whipping cream.
5. Bake for 22 to 27 minutes or until the sauce is piping hot and thickened.
6. Serve while hot.

LEMONY AND GARLICKY CHICKEN WINGS

Time: 25 mins | Serves 4
Net carbs: 1.8g | Fat: 7.8g
Protein: 13.4g | Kcal: 131

INGREDIENTS

- 8 chicken wings
- 1 tablespoon ghee, melted
- 2 garlic cloves, minced
- 60g leeks, chopped
- 2 tablespoons lemon juice
- 1 teaspoon Mediterranean spice mix

INSTRUCTIONS

1. Place all ingredients in a ceramic dish.
2. Cover and let it sit in your refrigerator for 2 hours.
3. Brush the chicken wings with melted ghee.
4. Grill the chicken wings for 15 to 20 minutes, turning them occasionally to ensure even cooking.
5. Serve while hot.

CHICKEN BREASTS IN CREAMY MUSHROOM SAUCE

Time: 15 mins | Serves 4
Net carbs: 4.3g | Fat: 20.8g
Protein: 30.9g | Kcal: 335

INGREDIENTS

- 2 chicken breast, skinless and boneless, cut into bite-sized pieces
- 2 garlic cloves, pressed
- 1 tablespoon olive oil
- 1 yellow onion, chopped
- 125ml cream of mushroom soup

INSTRUCTIONS

1 Heat the olive oil in a nonstick skillet over medium-high flame.
2 Once hot, cook the onion for about 4 minutes or until caramelized and softened.
3 Cook the garlic for 30 seconds more.
4 Sear the chicken breast for approximately 5 minutes, stirring continuously to ensure even cooking. Pour in the cream of mushroom soup.
5 Turn the heat to a simmer and continue to cook for about 8 minutes until the sauce has reduced and thickened.
6 Serve warm chicken topped with the sauce.

PORK WITH DIJON SAUCE

Time: 20 mins | Serves 4

Net carbs: 5.4g | Fat: 17.5g

Protein: 40g | Kcal: 343

INGREDIENTS

- 500g pork fillets
- 2 scallions, chopped
- 2 cloves garlic, minced
- 125ml water or dry white wine
- 2 tablespoons whole-grain Dijon mustard

INSTRUCTIONS

1 Melt 2 tablespoons of butter in a nonstick skillet over a moderate flame.

2 Sear the pork for 3 to 4 minutes per side and set aside.

3 Sauté the scallions and garlic in the pan drippings for 1 to 2 minutes.

4 Pour in water or white wine to scrape up the browned bits that stick to the bottom of the skillet.

5 Add in Dijon mustard along with the pork.

6 Partially cover and cook for a further 12 minutes or until the sauce has reduced by half.

7 Serve the pork fillets garnished with the sauce.

EASY ROASTED PORK SHOULDER

Time: 4 hours | Serves 4

Net carbs: 0.6g | Fat: 40.1g

Protein: 57g | Kcal: 609

INGREDIENTS

- 1kg pork shoulder
- 2 tablespoons coconut aminos
- 125ml water or red wine
- 1 tablespoon Dijon mustard
- 1 tablespoon Mediterranean spice mix

INSTRUCTIONS

1 Place the ingredients in a ceramic dish.
2 Allow it to marinate in the refrigerator for at least 2 hours.
3 Put the rack into a roasting pan, then lower the marinated pork onto the rack.
4 Roast in the preheated oven at 210 degrees Celsius for 30 minutes.
5 Turn the heat to 170 degrees.
6 Continue to roast an additional 3 hours, basting with the marinade.
7 Serve while hot.

MUSTARD PORK ROAST

Time: 1 hour | Serves 5

Net carbs: 0.1g | Fat: 20.1g

Protein: 48g | Kcal: 386

INGREDIENTS

- ◆ 1 ½ tablespoons olive oil
- ◆ 1kg pork loin roast, trimmed
- ◆ 1 tablespoon pork rub seasoning blend
- ◆ 1 tablespoon stone-ground mustard
- ◆ 1 tablespoon fresh lemon juice

INSTRUCTIONS

1   Massage the pork with olive oil on all sides.
2   Spread the pork rub seasoning blend, mustard, and lemon juice all over the roast.
3   Grill the pork over indirect heat for about 55 minutes or so or until cooked through.

WHITE SEA BASS CHOWDER

Time: 20 mins | Serves 4
Net carbs: 3.8g | Fat: 17.8g
Protein: 21.3g | Kcal: 257

INGREDIENTS

- 375g sea bass, broken into chunks
- 2 teaspoons butter, at room temperature
- 230g double cream
- 1/2 white onion, chopped
- 1 tablespoon fish seasoning

INSTRUCTIONS

1. In a soup pot, melt the butter over medium-high heat.
2. Sauté the onion until just tender.
3. Stir in Fish seasoning along with 750ml of water; bring to a boil.
4. Turn the heat to medium-low and allow it to simmer for about 10 minutes.
5. Stir in the sea bass and double cream.
6. Continue to simmer for about 5 minutes until cooked through.
7. Serve in individual bowls.

CLASSIC FISH CURRY

Time: 20 mins | Serves 4
Net carbs: 3.1g | Fat: 6.9g
Protein: 34.8g | Kcal: 226

INGREDIENTS

- 1.5kg tilapia
- 1 tablespoon peanut oil
- 1 shallot, chopped
- 1 tablespoon curry paste
- 225g tomato onion sauce
- 250ml chicken broth

INSTRUCTIONS

1 Heat the peanut oil in a wok over medium-high heat.
2 Cook the shallot for 2 to 3 minutes until tender and fragrant.
3 Pour in tomato onion sauce along with the chicken broth.
4 Bring to a boil.
5 Reduce the heat to a simmer and stir in the curry paste and tilapia.
6 Season with salt and pepper to your liking.
7 Continue to simmer, partially covered, for 10 to 12 minutes until heated through.
8 Serve while hot.

HADDOCK AND PARMESAN FISH BURGERS

Time: 20 mins | Serves 4
Net carbs: 1.5g | Fat: 11.4g
Protein: 15.4g | Kcal: 174

INGREDIENTS

- 240g smoked haddock
- 4 lemon wedges
- 1 egg
- 25g scallions, chopped
- 25g Parmesan cheese, grated

INSTRUCTIONS

1 Heat 1 tablespoon of olive oil in a frying pan over medium-high flame.
2 Once hot, cook the haddock for 5 to 6 minutes.
3 Flake the fish with a fork, discarding the skin and bones.
4 Add in cheese, eggs, and scallions; season with sea salt and pepper to taste.
5 Heat 1 tablespoon of olive oil until sizzling.
6 Fry your burgers for 5 to 6 minutes until they are thoroughly cooked.
7 Garnish with lemon wedges and serve.

BUTTERY STEAK WITH BROCCOLI

Time: 15 mins | Serves 3
Net carbs: 4.5g | Fat: 24.7g
Protein: 24.1g | Kcal: 331

INGREDIENTS

- 2 tablespoons butter, room temperature
- 250g broccoli, cut into florets
- 70g steak marinade
- 250g steak, sliced into pieces
- 50g scallions, chopped

INSTRUCTIONS

1. Place the steak marinade and beef in a ceramic bowl.
2. Let it marinate in your refrigerator for 3 hours.
3. In a frying pan, melt 1 tablespoon of butter over medium-high heat.
4. Sauté the broccoli for 2 to 3 minutes or until it is crisp-tender, then set aside.
5. Heat the remaining tablespoon of butter in the pan.
6. Sauté the scallions until tender for 2 to 3 minutes, then set aside.
7. Brown the steak, adding a small amount of the reserved marinade.
8. Stir in the reserved vegetables and continue to cook until everything is thoroughly warmed. Serve while hot.

AROMATIC BEEF STEW

Time: 55 mins | Serves 6
Net carbs: 2.7g | Fat: 21.5g
Protein: 17.4g | Kcal: 277

INGREDIENTS

- ◆ 1.5kg beef steak, cut into bite-sized cubes
- ◆ 25g onions, chopped
- ◆ 2 Italian peppers, chopped
- ◆ 1 celery stalk, chopped
- ◆ 270g tomato sauce with garlic

INSTRUCTIONS

1. In a heavy-bottomed pot, melt 1 teaspoon of lard over medium-high heat.
2. Sear the beef for about 10 minutes until brown, then set aside.
3. In the pan drippings, sauté the onion, Italian peppers, and celery for 5 to 6 minutes until they have softened.
4. Return the beef to the pot along with tomato sauce.
5. Season with salt and black pepper.
6. Let it simmer, partially covered, for 35 to 40 minutes.
7. Serve while hot.

SNACKS & DESSERTS

CHEESY CHICKEN ROLLS

Time: 30 mins | Serves 5
Net carbs: 7.2g | Fat: 11.1g
Protein: 36.8g | Kcal: 289

INGREDIENTS

- 5 slices ham
- 5 chicken fillets, about 0.6 cm thin
- 90g Ricotta cheese
- 30g cheddar cheese, grated
- 5g spicy tomato sauce

INSTRUCTIONS

1   Preheat the oven to 190 degrees Celsius.
2   Lay a slice of ham on each chicken fillet.
3   Mix Ricotta cheese and cheddar until well combined.
4   Spoon the cheese mixture onto the chicken fillets.
5   Roll them up, wrap in a piece of foil and place them in a lightly greased baking pan.
6   Bake in the preheated oven for approximately 15 minutes.
7   Flip them over, pour in tomato sauce and bake for another 15 minutes.
8   Serve while hot.

MOZZARELLA STUFFED MEATBALLS

Time: 25 mins | Serves 8

Net carbs: 1.6g | Fat: 31.3g

Protein: 23.8g | Kcal: 389

INGREDIENTS

- 750g minced pork
- 120g mozzarella string cheese, cubed
- 1 ripe tomato, pureed
- 1 garlic clove, minced
- 2 tablespoons shallots, chopped

INSTRUCTIONS

1 Mix minced pork, garlic, shallots, and tomato until well combined.

2 Take a tablespoon of the meat mixture and place a piece of the cheese inside.

3 Shape the meat around the cheese in a ball.

4 Repeat with the remaining ingredients.

5 Bake the meatballs in the preheated oven at 180 degrees Celsius for about 20 minutes.

6 Serve while hot.

HOT SAUCY RIBS

Time: 2 hours | Serves 4
Net carbs: 6.5g | Fat: 27g
Protein: 48.7g | Kcal: 472

INGREDIENTS

- 1kg spare ribs
- 1 teaspoon Dijon mustard
- 1 tablespoon rice wine
- 1 tablespoon avocado oil
- 500g spicy tomato sauce with garlic, no sugar added

INSTRUCTIONS

1   Preheat the oven to 180 degrees Celsius.
2   Toss the ribs with mustard, rice wine, and avocado oil.
3   Season with salt and pepper to taste.
4   Place the spare ribs on a foil-lined baking pan.
5   Bake in the preheated oven for 55 to 60 minutes.
6   Flip them over and roast for a further 55 minutes.
7   After that, pour the hot sauce over the ribs.
8   Place under the broiler for about 8 minutes.
9   Brush hot sauce onto each rib and serve immediately.

FAVOURITE BLT CUPS

Time: 15 mins | Serves 10

Net carbs: 1.6g | Fat: 8.3g

Protein: 2.7g | Kcal: 92

INGREDIENTS

- 10 pieces lettuce
- 10 tomatoes cherry tomatoes, discard the insides
- 2 tablespoons mayonnaise
- 5 tablespoons Parmigiano-Reggiano cheese, grated
- 150g bacon, chopped

INSTRUCTIONS

1 Cook the bacon in the preheated frying pan for about 6 minutes, then set aside.
2 In a mixing bowl, combine the mayonnaise and cheese.
3 Season with salt and black pepper to taste.
4 Divide the mixture between cherry tomatoes.
5 Top with the bacon.
6 Place on lettuce leaves and serve on a nice serving platter.

TURKEY ROLL-UPS WITH AVOCADO AND CHEESE

Time: 10 mins | Serves 8
Net carbs: 7g | Fat: 23.9g
Protein: 22.4g | Kcal: 332

INGREDIENTS

◆ 16 slices cooked turkey breasts

◆ 1/2 fresh lemon, juiced

◆ Salt and black pepper, to taste

◆ 16 slices Swiss cheese

◆ 2 avocados, pitted, peeled and diced

INSTRUCTIONS

1 Drizzle fresh lemon juice over diced avocado.
2 Divide avocado pieces among turkey slices.
3 Season with salt and black pepper.
4 Add the slice of Swiss cheese to each roll.
5 Roll them up and serve immediately.

BEST KETO SUSHI

Time: 15 mins | Serves 8

Net carbs: 3.4g | Fat: 37.2g

Protein: 1.5g | Kcal: 350

INGREDIENTS

◆ 8 bacon slices

◆ 2 scallions, finely chopped

◆ 1 avocado, mashed

◆ 2 tablespoons fresh lemon juice

◆ 120g cream cheese, softened

INSTRUCTIONS

1 Thoroughly combine the scallions, cream cheese, avocado, and fresh lemon juice.
2 Divide the mixture between the bacon slices.
3 Roll them up, secure them with toothpicks, and serve.

PRAWN COCKTAIL SKEWERS

Time: 15 mins | Serves 4
Net carbs: 5.1g | Fat: 8.3g
Protein: 20.4g | Kcal: 179

INGREDIENTS

- 500g king prawns, deveined and cleaned
- 2 tablespoons fresh lime juice
- 150g cherry tomatoes
- 2 bell peppers, diced
- 2 tablespoons olive oil

INSTRUCTIONS

1. In a large saucepan, heat olive oil over medium-high heat.
2. Sauté the prawns for 3 to 4 minutes until they are pink.
3. Stir in Cajun seasoning mix.
4. Toss king prawns with the lime juice.
5. Thread the prawns, cherry tomatoes and peppers onto bamboo skewers.
6. Serve immediately.

RESTAURANT-STYLE ONIONS RINGS

Time: 20 mins | Serves 4
Net carbs: 5.7g | Fat: 27.8g
Protein: 10.1g | Kcal: 332

INGREDIENTS

- ◆ 65g coconut flour
- ◆ 3 eggs
- ◆ 2 onions, cut into 1/2-inch thick rings
- ◆ 120g pork rinds
- ◆ 90g parmesan cheese, grated

INSTRUCTIONS

1. Place the coconut flour in a shallow bowl.
2. In a separate shallow bowl, mix the eggs and gradually add in 4 tablespoons of water.
3. In the third bowl, mix the pork rinds and parmesan.
4. Dip the onion rings into the coconut flour.
5. Submerge them into the egg mixture.
6. Press the onion rings in the parmesan mixture.
7. Place the onion rings on a lightly greased baking rack and bake at 210 degrees Celsius for about 15 minutes.
8. Serve while hot.

SPICY CHICKEN DRUMSTICKS

Time: 25 mins | Serves 6
Net carbs: 2.3g | Fat: 2.5g
Protein: 34.2g | Kcal: 179

INGREDIENTS

- 1kg chicken drumsticks
- 70g hot sauce
- 1 teaspoon garlic powder
- 1 teaspoon dried oregano
- 1 tablespoon stone-ground mustard

INSTRUCTIONS

1. Start by preheating your oven to 210 degrees Celsius.
2. Sprinkle chicken drumettes with oregano; season with salt and black pepper.
3. Brush chicken drumettes with nonstick cooking oil and bake in the preheated oven for about 20 minutes.
4. Toss chicken drumettes with hot sauce, mustard and garlic powder.
5. Place them under the preheated broiler for 5 to 6 minutes or until they are golden brown.
6. Serve while hot.

RANCH KALE CRISPS

Time: 15 mins | Serves 4
Net carbs: 1.4g | Fat: 6.6g
Protein: 0.6g | Kcal: 68

INGREDIENTS

- 2 tablespoons olive oil
- 280g kale, torn into pieces
- Sea salt, to taste
- 2 teaspoon Ranch seasoning mix

INSTRUCTIONS

1 Preheat the oven to 150 degrees Celsius.
2 Toss the kale leaves with olive oil, salt, and Ranch seasoning mix until well coated.
3 Bake for about 12 minutes and let it cool before storing, then serve.

CHEWY CHOCOLATE CHIP COOKIES

Time: 10 mins | Serves 10
Net carbs: 4.1g | Fat: 9.5g
Protein: 2.1g | Kcal: 104

INGREDIENTS

- 65g almond flour
- 4 tablespoons double cream
- 80g sugar-free chocolate chips
- 5g coconut, unsweetened and shredded
- 175g fruit syrup

INSTRUCTIONS

1. In a mixing bowl, combine all of the above ingredients until well combined.
2. Shape the batter into bite-sized balls.
3. Flatten the balls using a fork or your hand.
4. Place in your refrigerator until ready to serve.

LIGHT GREEK CHEESECAKE

Time: 1.5 hours | Serves 6
Net carbs: 6.9g | Fat: 45g
Protein: 11.5g | Kcal: 471

INGREDIENTS

- 300g whipped Greek yoghurt cream cheese
- 6 tablespoons butter, melted
- 25g sweetener
- 2 eggs
- 200g almond flour

INSTRUCTIONS

1 Preheat the oven to 160 degrees Celsius.
2 Combine the almond flour and butter and press the crust into a lightly buttered springform pan.
3 Beat the Greek-style yoghurt with the sweetener until everything is well mixed.
4 Fold in the eggs, one at a time, and mix well to make sure that everything is combined well.
5 Pour the filling over the crust.
6 Bake in the preheated oven for about 35 minutes until the middle is still jiggly.
7 Serve once cooled and set.

EASY ALMOND FUDGE BARS

Time: 5 mins | Serves 7
Net carbs: 4.7g | Fat: 6.8g
Protein: 0.5g | Kcal: 78

INGREDIENTS

- 3 tablespoons coconut oil
- 25g sweetener
- 4 tablespoons coconut flakes
- 4 tablespoons cacao powder, no sugar added
- 130g almonds

INSTRUCTIONS

1 Line a baking pan with wax paper.
2 Blend all ingredients in your food processor until everything is well incorporated.
3 Scrape down the sides with a rubber spatula.
4 Press firmly into the prepared pan and freeze for 10 minutes or until firm enough to slice.
5 Cut into squares.
6 Store leftovers in the refrigerator or freezer.

BASIC KETO BROWNIES

Time: 1 hour | Serves 10
Net carbs: 5.4g | Fat: 19.5g
Protein: 4.7g | Kcal: 205

INGREDIENTS

- 110g coconut oil
- 90g baking chocolate, unsweetened
- 5 tablespoons coconut flour
- 60g cocoa powder, unsweetened
- ½ teaspoon baking powder
- 4 eggs

INSTRUCTIONS

1   Preheat the oven to 160 degrees Celsius.
2   Thoroughly combine the coconut flour and cocoa powder.
3   Add in ½ teaspoon of baking powder.
4   Whisk the eggs with a keto sweetener, of choice.
5   Add in the melted coconut oil and chocolate.
6   Gradually stir the dry ingredients into the egg mixture, whisking constantly.
7   Scrape the batter into a buttered baking pan.
8   Bake in the preheated oven for 45 to 50 minutes or until a tester inserted into the middle of your brownie comes out dry.
9   Serve once cooled.

AUTUMN KETO CREPES

Time: 15 mins | Serves 6
Net carbs: 6.9g | Fat: 21.7g
Protein: 11.6g | Kcal: 260

INGREDIENTS

- 4 tablespoons pumpkin puree, sugar-free
- 4 eggs
- 180g ricotta cheese, at room temperature
- 100g almond flour
- 60g pecans, fine ground

INSTRUCTIONS

1 Combine almond flour and pecans along with 1/2 teaspoon of baking powder.
2 Add in the eggs, one at a time, whisking after each addition.
3 Add in ricotta cheese and pumpkin puree.
4 Mix again to combine well.
5 In a lightly greased pan, cook your pancakes for about 3 minutes on each side.
6 Serve with favourite keto toppings.

PEANUT BUTTER BALLS

Time: 35 mins | Serves 10
Net carbs: 7.5g | Fat: 23.2g
Protein: 9.9g | Kcal: 275

INGREDIENTS

- ◆ 1/4 teaspoon ground cinnamon
- ◆ 100g sweetener
- ◆ 180g chunky peanut butter
- ◆ 110g peanuts, finely chopped
- ◆ 180g chocolate, sugar-free, chopped

INSTRUCTIONS

1 Mix all ingredients until smooth.
2 Place the batter in your refrigerator for 30 minutes or until firm enough to handle.
3 Shape the batter into bite-sized balls and place in your refrigerator until ready to serve.

SMOOTHIE BOWL WITH RASPBERRIES

Time: 5 mins | Serves 2
Net carbs: 6.5g | Fat: 4.9g
Protein: 4.2g | Kcal: 90

INGREDIENTS

- ◆ ½ teaspoon vanilla extract
- ◆ 2 tablespoon cacao nibs, sugar-free
- ◆ ⅓ cup raspberries
- ◆ 250ml almond milk
- ◆ 1 teaspoon sweetener

INSTRUCTIONS

1 Blend the almond milk, sweetener, vanilla, and raspberries until creamy, smooth, and uniform.
2 Pour into the prepared bowl and top with cacao nibs.

VELVETY COCONUT CHEESECAKE

Time: 30 mins | Serves 6
Net carbs: 4.9g | Fat: 22.5g
Protein: 6.1g | Kcal: 236

INGREDIENTS

- 60g coconut flour
- 180g mascarpone cheese, at room temperature
- 120g heavy whipping cream
- 2 tablespoons cocoa powder
- 5 tablespoons coconut oil

INSTRUCTIONS

1 Combine coconut flour, cocoa powder, and 3 tablespoons of coconut oil.
2 Add keto sweetener to taste.
3 Press the crust into a lightly-oiled baking pan.
4 Then, mix mascarpone cheese and 2 tablespoons of coconut oil in your microwave.
5 Spread the filling over the crust.
6 Top with heavy whipping cream.
7 Place in your refrigerator until ready to serve.

EASY MOLTEN CAKE

Time: 20 mins | Serves 4
Net carbs: 7.6g | Fat: 45g
Protein: 10.6g | Kcal: 478

INGREDIENTS

- 90g bakers' chocolate, sugar-free
- 4 eggs
- 1 tablespoon unsweetened cocoa powder
- 120g butter
- 2 tablespoons almond meal

INSTRUCTIONS

1   Start by preheating your oven to 190 degrees Celsius.
2   Pour 2 cups of water into a baking dish.
3   Beat the eggs and butter until well mixed.
4   Melt the chocolate and add the melted chocolate to the mixing bowl.
5   Fold in the almond meal and cocoa powder; add in sweetener to taste.
6   Spoon the mixture into four buttered ramekins.
7   Place the ramekins into the baking dish. Bake in the preheated for 10 to 12 minutes.
8   Invert each cake onto a serving plate.

FLAX SEED AND PECAN PORRIDGE

Time: 10 mins | Serves 2

Net carbs: 6.7g | Fat: 32g

Protein: 4.8g | Kcal: 327

INGREDIENTS

- 125ml canned coconut milk
- 2 tablespoons golden flaxseeds, ground
- A few drops of liquid sweetener
- 2 tablespoons pecans, ground
- 2 tablespoons coconut flour

INSTRUCTIONS

1 In a saucepan, bring 190ml of water and coconut milk to a boil.
2 Add in pecans, coconut flour, golden flaxseeds, and liquid sweetener.
3 Reduce the heat to medium-low.
4 Continue to simmer for 2 to 3 minutes or until slightly thickened.
5 Serve well-chilled.

BONUS: 14-DAY KETO DIET WEIGHT LOSS PLANNER

Day 1

Breakfast: Famous Double-Cheese Chips

> Time: 10 mins | Serves 6
> Net carbs: 1.1g | Fat: 11.7g
> Protein: 9.4g | Kcal: 148

INGREDIENTS

- 70g Parmesan cheese, shredded
- 1 tablespoon Italian seasoning blend
- 85g Grana Padano cheese, shredded

INSTRUCTIONS

1 Start by preheating your oven to 180 degrees Celsius.
2 Mix the ingredients in a bowl.
3 Spoon tablespoon-sized heaps of the mixture onto foil-lined baking sheets.
4 Bake in the preheated oven for approximately 7 minutes until they are browned around the edges.
5 Transfer the cheese chips to paper towels and allow them to cool until crisp, then serve.

Lunch: Classic Family Cheeseburgers (See page 36)

Dinner: Spaghetti Bolognese (See page 52)

Day 2

Breakfast: Hard-Boiled Eggs with Avocado (See page 15)

Lunch: Sea Bass with Dill Sauce

> Time: 25 mins | Serves 4
> Net carbs: 6.2g | Fat: 17g
> Protein: 43.2g | Kcal: 374

INGREDIENTS

- 70g Greek yoghurt
- 1 tablespoon fresh dill, chopped
- 1kg sea bass fillets
- 50g red onions, sliced
- 2 bell peppers, deveined and sliced

INSTRUCTIONS

1   Start by preheating your oven to 200 degrees Celsius.
2   Toss sea bass fillets, bell peppers, and onions with 1 tablespoon of olive oil.
3   Season with salt and pepper.
4   Place the fish and vegetables in a lightly greased baking dish.
5   Bake for 20 to 22 minutes, rotating the pan once or twice.
6   Make the sauce by whisking Greek yoghurt and chopped dill.
7   Serve warm fish and vegetables with the sauce on the side.

Dinner: Hearty Beef and Vegetable Stew (See page 53)

DAY 3

Breakfast: Breakfast Egg Salad (See page 20)
Lunch: Chicken Thigh Salad (See page 37)
Dinner: Beef with Harvest Vegetables

Time: 20 mins | Serves 5

Net carbs: 4g | Fat: 14.3g

Protein: 30.1g | Kcal: 261

INGREDIENTS

- 2 tablespoons olive oil
- 750g beef steak, cut into bite-sized cubes
- 2 bell peppers, deveined and sliced
- 140g cauliflower florets
- 1 red onion, sliced

INSTRUCTIONS

1 In a saucepan, heat the olive oil over medium-high flame.
2 Sear the beef for 4 to 5 minutes until no longer pink, then set aside.
3 Cook the peppers, cauliflower, and onion in the pan drippings until tender, adding about 60ml of water if needed.
4 Bring to a boil and immediately reduce the heat to medium-low.
5 Simmer for 10 minutes or until the cooking liquid has evaporated.

Day 4

Breakfast: Egg Cups with Ham

Time: 30 mins | Serves 6

Net carbs: 2.8g | Fat: 19.1g

Protein: 17.5g | Kcal: 258

INGREDIENTS

- 6 thin slices of ham
- 6 eggs
- 120g cream cheese
- 1 teaspoon mustard
- 180g cheddar cheese, shredded

INSTRUCTIONS

1 Line muffin cups with cupcake liners.
2 Add a ham slice to each muffin cup and gently press down.
3 In a mixing dish, whisk the eggs, cream cheese, and mustard.
4 Season with salt and pepper to taste.
5 Spoon the egg mixture into the cups.
6 Top with the shredded cheese.
7 Bake in the preheated oven at 180 degrees Celsius for approximately 27 minutes.
8 Garnish with 2 tablespoons of green onions just before serving and enjoy!

Lunch: Fajita with Zucchini (See page 38)

Dinner: Classic Sunday Roast (See page 55)

Day 5

Breakfast: Skinny Eggs with Spinach (See page 21)

Lunch: Easy Moroccan Tajine

> Time: 50 mins | Serves 4
>
> Net carbs: 3.5g | Fat: 12.9g
>
> Protein: 7.6g | Kcal: 155

INGREDIENTS

- ◆ 2 tablespoons leeks, sliced
- ◆ 250g zucchini, thinly sliced
- ◆ 120g cheddar cheese, grated
- ◆ 60g heavy cream
- ◆ 1 tablespoon Moroccan spice mix

INSTRUCTIONS

1   Brush the sides and bottom of a baking dish with 1 tablespoon of melted butter.
2   Place 125g of the zucchini slices in the bottom of the baking dish.
3   Add 1 tablespoon of leeks.
4   Sprinkle with the Moroccan spice mix.
5   Top with the cheddar cheese.
6   Repeat the layers of zucchini and leeks.
7   In a mixing bowl, thoroughly combine cheddar cheese and heavy cream.
8   Spoon the mixture over the vegetable layer.
9   Bake in the preheated oven at 190 degrees Celsius for approximately 45 minutes until the top is nicely browned.
10 Serve while hot.

Dinner: Cheesy Zucchini Lasagna (See page 56)

DAY 6

Breakfast: Frittata with Mediterranean Herbs (See page 22)
Lunch: Spicy Pork Meatballs (See page 39)
Dinner: Double Cheese Italian Chicken

Time: 20 mins | Serves 2
Net carbs: 5.8g | Fat: 46g
Protein: 37.5g | Kcal: 589

INGREDIENTS

- ◆ 2 chicken drumsticks
- ◆ 150ml chicken bone broth
- ◆ 60g baby spinach
- ◆ 1 teaspoon Italian spice mix
- ◆ 115g cream cheese
- ◆ 235g Grana Padano cheese, grated

INSTRUCTIONS

1. In a saucepan, heat 1 tablespoon of oil over medium-high heat.
2. Sear the chicken drumsticks for 7 to 8 minutes or until nicely browned on all sides and set aside.
3. Pour in chicken bone broth.
4. Add in spinach and continue to cook for 5 minutes more until spinach has wilted.
5. Add in the Italian spice mix, cream cheese, Asiago cheese, and reserved chicken drumsticks. Partially cover and continue to cook for 5 more minutes.
6. Serve while warm.

Day 7

Breakfast: Cheese Stuffed Peppers

Time: 25 mins | Serves 4

Net carbs: 6.4g | Fat: 9.8g

Protein: 7.8g | Kcal: 140

INGREDIENTS

- 4 summer bell peppers, divined and halved
- 60g mozzarella cheese, crumbled
- 2 tablespoons Greek-style yoghurt
- 120g cream cheese
- 1 clove garlic, minced

INSTRUCTIONS

1. Boil the peppers until they are just tender.
2. Thoroughly combine the cheese, yoghurt, and garlic.
3. Stuff your peppers with this filling.
4. Place the stuffed peppers in a foil-lined baking dish.
5. Bake in the preheated oven at 180 degrees Celsius for about 10 minutes.
6. Serve while hot.

Lunch: Autumn Butternut Squash Stew (See page 40)

Dinner: Easy Chicken Casserole (See page 58)

Day 8

Breakfast: Classic Keto Muffins (See page 25)

Lunch: Herbed Pork Meatloaf

Time: 1 hour | Serves 6

Net carbs: 2.8g | Fat: 23.1g

Protein: 30g | Kcal: 344

INGREDIENTS

- 750g minced pork
- 50g scallions, chopped
- 40g flaxseed meal
- 2 eggs, beaten
- 90g herbed tomato sauce

INSTRUCTIONS

1. Preheat an oven to 180 degrees Celsius.
2. Brush the sides and bottom of a baking pan with nonstick cooking spray.
3. Mix the minced pork, scallions, flaxseed meal, and eggs in a bowl.
4. Mix until everything is well incorporated.
5. Spoon the meatloaf mixture into the greased pan and bake for 30 minutes.
6. Spread the herbed tomato sauce on top of the meatloaf.
7. Bake for a further 25 to 28 minutes.
8. Serve while hot.

Dinner: Lemony and Garlicky Chicken Wings (See page 59)

DAY 9

Breakfast: Breakfast Sausage and Cheese Bites (See page 23)

Lunch: Fried Cod Fillets (See page 41)

Dinner: Easy Beef Ragù

Time: 25 mins | Serves 6

Net carbs: 4.9g | Fat: 21.8g

Protein: 34g | Kcal: 349

INGREDIENTS

- 750g minced beef
- 285ml beef bone broth
- 1 celery rib, chopped
- 1 bell pepper, deseeded and chopped
- 450g tomato sauce with garlic, no sugar added

INSTRUCTIONS

1 Cook minced beef in a lightly greased pot for 5 to 6 minutes until no longer pink, then set aside.
2 In the pan drippings, cook the celery and the peppers until they are tender.
3 Stir in the tomato sauce and beef bone broth.
4 Season with Italian herb mix and bring to a boil.
5 Reduce heat to medium-low and add the reserved beef to the pot.
6 Continue to cook until the sauce has reduced by half.
7 Serve while hot.

DAY 10

Breakfast: Creamy Dilled Egg Salad

Time: 20 mins | Serves 3

Net carbs: 0.9g | Fat: 19.4g

Protein: 7.6g | Kcal: 212

INGREDIENTS

- ◆ 4 eggs, peeled and chopped
- ◆ 1 scallion, chopped
- ◆ 1 tablespoon fresh dill minced
- ◆ 1 teaspoon Dijon mustard
- ◆ 4 tablespoons mayonnaise

INSTRUCTIONS

1. Add the eggs and water to a saucepan and bring to a boil.
2. Remove from heat.
3. Allow the eggs to sit, covered, for about 11 minutes.
4. Peel and rinse the eggs under running water.
5. Chop the eggs and transfer them to a salad bowl.
6. Stir in the scallions, dill, mustard, and mayonnaise.
7. Taste and season with salt and pepper.

Lunch: Eggplant and Goat Cheese Bake (See page 42)

Dinner: Chicken Breasts in Creamy Mushroom Sauce (See page 60)

Day 11

Breakfast: Soufflé with Sausage and Cheese (See page 24)

Lunch: Kid-Friendly Sloppy Joes

Time: 45 mins | Serves 8

Net carbs: 2.6g | Fat: 16g

Protein: 22.7g | Kcal: 248

INGREDIENTS

- 1kg minced beef
- 1 teaspoon garlic, minced
- 1 shallot, chopped
- 1 Italian pepper, chopped
- 10g marinara sauce
- 8 keto buns

INSTRUCTIONS

1 Heat 2 tablespoons of olive oil in a nonstick skillet over moderate heat.
2 Cook the minced beef for 5 to 6 minutes, crumbling with a fork or wooden spatula.
3 Add in the shallot and continue to sauté for 3 to 4 minutes or until tender.
4 Stir in marinara sauce, Italian pepper, and garlic.
5 Bring to a rolling boil.
6 Reduce the heat to medium-low and partially cover.
7 Continue to simmer for 30 minutes longer.
8 Serve on keto buns.

Dinner: Pork with Dijon Sauce (See page 61)

Day 12

Breakfast: Breakfast Bacon and Kale Muffins (See page 26)
Lunch: Roasted Asparagus Salad (See page 43)
Dinner: Home-Style Chicken Kebab

> Time: 20 mins | Serves 2
> Net carbs: 6.2g | Fat: 23.2g
> Protein: 61g | Kcal: 498

INGREDIENTS

- ◆ 2 Roma tomatoes, chopped
- ◆ 500g chicken thighs, boneless, skinless and halved
- ◆ 2 tablespoons olive oil
- ◆ 125g Greek-style yoghurt
- ◆ 75g Swiss cheese, sliced

INSTRUCTIONS

1   Place the chicken thighs, yoghurt, tomatoes, and olive oil in a glass storage container.

2   Cover tightly and allow it to marinate in the refrigerator for 3 to 4 hours.

3   Thread the chicken thighs onto skewers, creating a thick log shape.

4   Grill the kebabs over medium-high heat for 3 or 4 minutes on each side.

5   Top with the cheese.

6   Continue to cook for 4 minutes or until the cheese is melted.

7   Serve while hot.

Day 13

Breakfast: Herbed Cheese Ball

Time: 10 mins | Serves 10
Net carbs: 2g | Fat: 15.7g
Protein: 7.2g | Kcal: 176

INGREDIENTS

- ◆ 125g sour cream
- ◆ 240g extra-sharp cheddar cheese, shredded
- ◆ 180g cream cheese, softened
- ◆ 2 tablespoons mayonnaise
- ◆ 1 tablespoon Moroccan herb mix

INSTRUCTIONS

1 Thoroughly combine sour cream, cheddar cheese, cream cheese, and mayonnaise.
2 Cover the mixture with plastic wrap and place it in your refrigerator for about 3 hours.
3 Roll the mixture over Moroccan herb mix until well coated.
4 Serve with assorted keto veggies.

Lunch: Anchovies with Caesar Dressing (See page 44)

Dinner: Easy Roasted Pork Shoulder (See page 62)

Day 14

Breakfast: Cheesy Mini Frittatas with Sausage (See page 27)
Lunch: Fish and Egg Salad (See page 45)
Dinner: Cod with Mustard Greens

Time: 20 mins | Serves 4
Net carbs: 4.8g | Fat: 7.8g
Protein: 20.3g | Kcal: 171

INGREDIENTS

- 1 tablespoon olive oil
- 2 stalks green onions, sliced
- 260g vegetable broth
- 1 bell pepper, seeded and sliced
- 4 cod fish fillets
- 60g mustard greens, torn into bite-sized pieces

INSTRUCTIONS

1 Heat the oil in a saucepan over moderate heat.
2 Sauté green onions and peppers for about 4 minutes until they have softened.
3 Pour in vegetable broth.
4 Add in fish fillets along with salt and pepper to taste.
5 Fold in mustard greens.
6 Turn the temperature to simmer, cover, and continue to cook for about 12 minutes or until cooked through.
7 Serve while hot.

DISCLAIMER

This book contains opinions and ideas of the author and is meant to teach the reader informative and helpful knowledge while due care should be taken by the user in the application of the information provided. The instructions and strategies are possibly not right for every reader and there is no guarantee that they work for everyone. Using this book and implementing the information/recipes therein contained is explicitly your own responsibility and risk. This work with all its contents, does not guarantee correctness, completion, quality or correctness of the provided information. Misinformation or misprints cannot be completely eliminated.